WHY DO I HURT?

A PATIENT BOOK ABOUT THE NEUROSCIENCE F PAIN

Neuroscience Education
For Patients In Pain

Adriaan Louw
PT, PhD, CSMT

ISBN-978-0-9857186-2-6

Index

SCIENTIFIC SUPPORT FOR YOUR RECOVERY

In each section, you will notice some numbers in the sentences.
These numbers refer to scientific articles that support the
statements in your book. The details of each article are listed
at the back of your book.

⌐ The author of the book would like to offer
special thanks to the artist, Rod Bohner,
and the editor, Carolyn Raymond.

Introduction

Pain is a normal, human experience. Without the ability to experience pain, humans would not survive. Living in pain, however, is not normal. In the last several years, our knowledge of how pain works has increased considerably. In many persistent pain states, focus has been shifted to the nervous system and the brain as main contributors to pain.[1,2] This is for all pain, regardless of where it is in the body and how long it has been going on. A big reason why pain rates are increasing is the fact that too much focus has been placed on tissues, such as muscles, ligaments and joints, which generally are healed between three and six months.[3,4]

TISSUES HEAL

It's important to know that persistent pain is more due to the sensitive nervous system and how the brain processes information from the body and the environment.[5-7] This book was written to educate you on how the nervous system and the brain process information and contribute to your pain experience.

The latest research shows that the more you know about pain and how it works, the better off you'll be.[8] This includes moving and functioning better, experiencing less pain and having an increased ability and interest in doing more healthy exercise and movement.[8-10] This knowledge is essential in your recovery. Additionally, research has shown that anyone is able to understand the science of the nerves. So welcome to learning about this science of the nerves, which is more accurately called the neuroscience of pain.[11]

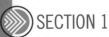# Your tissues and your nerves

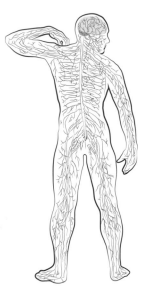

Because you're reading this book, you're undoubtedly experiencing pain somewhere in your body. This pain could be in one spot, such as an elbow or your back, a region of pain that might include several areas, or pain all over your body.

Each of your body areas where you're experiencing pain has nerves in and around them. This is normal. If someone kicks you in the leg or slaps your face, the nerves will let you know there's someone very unfriendly in your vicinity. Your body contains 45 miles of nerves and more than 400 individual nerves – all connected like a network of roads.[12,13] These nerves connect all body parts to the spinal cord so messages can be sent from your tissues to the brain for analysis.[5,6]

Your nerves monitor your body and inform you and your brain of anything going on in your body. Some nerves work like an alarm system. At any given time, all nerves have a little bit of electricity running through them. This is normal and shows you're alive.[5,6]

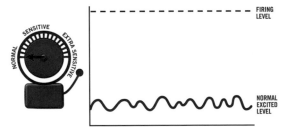

Consider the example of when you step on a nail. You want to know about it so you can remove it, get a tetanus shot and avoid an infection. The nerves in your foot need to send the message to your brain so that action can be taken. Nerves send messages by using electrical impulses. When there is danger, such as a nail in the foot, the nerves increase electrical activity and "wake up," sending a lot of danger messages to your spinal cord and ultimately to your brain. They let the brain know there is danger and action is required.[5,6]

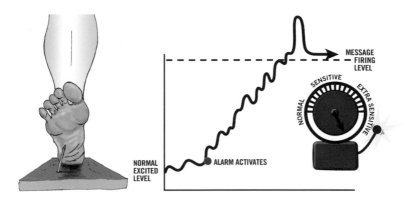

The brain's action may include walking funny, producing stress chemicals in your body or even using a choice word or two. In this case, it's logical for the brain to produce pain in your foot so that you are alerted to the nail and you take action, such as taking the nail out. Once you take care of the danger, the nail in this case, it also makes sense for the alarm system to settle down and return to its normal resting level of activity – ready for the next danger. You'll probably learn to avoid stepping on nails as well.

When you hurt yourself, have an accident, undergo surgery or experience a lot of emotional stress, the same process as the nail in the foot occurs. When you develop pain in a certain body part, the nerves in these areas "wake up," alerting your brain to the danger in the area. The nerves around the areas alert the spinal cord, which in turn tells the brain there is a problem in the area and action is possibly required.

THIS ALARM MAY CAUSE YOU TO DO THE FOLLOWING:
✓ See your family doctor
✓ See a physical therapist
✓ Get X-rays or an MRI
✓ Seek additional help

In essence, your nerves have done their job.

In some people, the nerves that "wake up" to alert you to the danger in your tissues calm down very slowly and remain elevated and "buzzing." In this state, it does not take much activity, such as sitting, reaching, bending or driving, to get the nerves to fire off danger messages to the brain. The nerves become extra sensitive.[5,6]

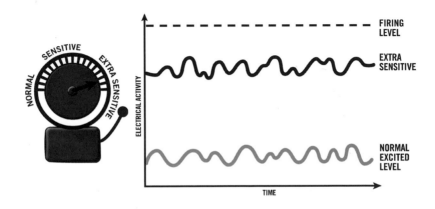

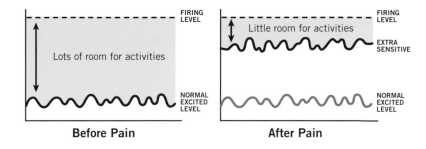

Before Pain	After Pain

This response is actually quite normal, but it impedes on movement and function a lot. Look at the two drawings shown above. Before you developed pain, you were able to perform any task quite easily and for long periods, such as driving, doing dishes, or working on a computer. But since you developed pain, you've noticed and reported it doesn't take but a few minutes of the same task to experience pain. No wonder you think something must be wrong! Think of the activities that you used to do such as exercising, washing loads of laundry, leading a meeting or cooking a meal. Now, think about how limited you are with the level of pain you now experience. The main issue is increased nerve sensitivity.[5-7]

Another way to think about your nerves is to compare them to your home alarm system.

At your house, imagine an alarm system is set up. Normal day-to-day activities do not set off the alarm. It's set to be sensitive to bigger issues, such as someone breaking a window. Since you have experienced pain, your alarm system is so sensitive that when a leaf blows by the house, it sets off the alarm. The system needs to be changed to decrease its sensitivity.

5

How do I know if my alarm system is set at *too sensitive*?[9,14]

This a great question. See if any of these answers fit your situation and mark them:

❏ Your activity level before reaching pain has decreased a lot.

❏ You instinctively know you have become more sensitive, or even over-sensitive.

❏ Pressure on your skin or around the painful area is very sensitive.

❏ When doctors and therapists test you or move your body parts, you are very sensitive.

❏ You are currently on medicine to calm your nerves, such as Cymbalta™, Lyrica™ and Neurontin™ or anti-depressants, such as Paxil™, Zoloft™ and Prozac™.

Why did my nerves stay sensitive? This didn't happen to my neighbor

As mentioned before, in some people nerves are slow to calm down. Why is this? You know that your neighbor, friend or family member had a similar injury or accident, yet they bounced right back. In some people, there are so many issues surrounding the pain experience that the brain decides it's best to keep the alarm system elevated.[15] For example:

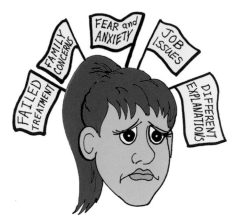

PAIN
Even though pain is a normal protective mechanism, the pain experience is stressful, and no fun. Shortly after an injury or accident, it's quite normal to experience pain. This pain will lead to an elevated alarm system to protect you.

DIFFERENT EXPLANATIONS FOR YOUR PAIN
You can feel more stressed when you're not sure about what treatment options you should follow and you have different explanations about what to expect. Everyone has an opinion, including family members, friends, doctors, therapists, Dr. Oz and the Internet. All this uncertainty will leave the alarm system elevated for a while as you seek the answers.

FAMILY AND JOB

Pain has and will continue to impact your family life and your job. This impact may include doctor and physical therapy visits, expensive tests, lost work time and frustration. In addition, you may have concerns about money, the future, or your ability to work. These concerns provide little incentive to your brain to turn the alarm system down.

FAILED TREATMENT

You may begin to wonder why the treatment isn't working or why the injections helped your neighbor, but not you. You may have attended countless doctors' visits, therapy visits and more, yet the pain isn't better. In fact, it may even be worse. As long as your brain asks these questions and has concerns, it will keep your alarm system elevated.

FEAR

Considering the failed treatments, various explanations for your pain, job issues and family concerns, there is bound to be a lot of uncertainty. The uncertainty is usually accompanied by some anxiety or fear. This is quite common, but it has been shown that fear of injury, or re-injury, and fear of exercise or movement will keep the alarm system turned on, rather than off.[16]

Your alarm system is even more complicated[5,6]

You may have noticed that even beyond the "normal" sensitivity described, you have become sensitive to other things, such as cold temperature and stress. Inside your nerves, there are various sensors also designed to protect and inform you of any changes in your life.[17,18] Various sensors have been identified, but the following may be of particular interest to you:

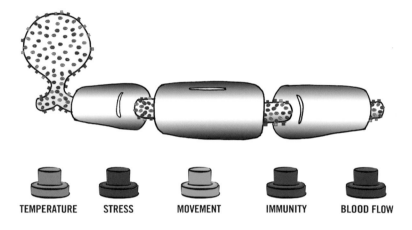

| TEMPERATURE | STRESS | MOVEMENT | IMMUNITY | BLOOD FLOW |

TEMPERATURE

There are sensors in nerves that tell you if there is a change in temperature. It is not uncommon to get sensitive to cold temperature and feel more aches and pains in the affected area when it gets cold out.

STRESS

There are sensors in nerves that are sensitive to stress chemicals flowing in your blood. The more stressed, anxious, nervous or upset you are, the more you will experience an increase in aches and pains. The more stress chemicals that run through your body, the more stress sensors are activated.

MOVEMENT AND PRESSURE

There are sensors in your nerves that are sensitive to movement and pressure around them. For example, movement after surgery or injury may activate a few more sensors and make the movement extra sensitive for a little while.

IMMUNITY

When you are sick, with the flu for example, there are many immune molecules floating through your body, helping you deal with the illness. This also happens following injury or surgery, with recent research showing that when you are really worried about an inflamed body part, you'll have an immune response. Nerves have sensors telling them of the increased immune molecules, and the immune chemicals produced can make you ache.

BLOOD FLOW

There are sensors in your nerves that are sensitive to the amount of blood around your tissues. When blood flow slows down slightly, after sitting too long for example, these sensors "wake up" and make the nerves sensitive.

Key points about nerve sensors:

✓ When you develop pain, your nerves increase their sensitivity to protect you.

✓ This is a normal response that happens in every human being.

✓ These sensors are constantly updated based on your environment.

Another way to view the sensors is to think of your car. Modern cars have sensors all over them to alert you to oil pressure, fuel, engine or other issues. Any of these could cause a dashboard light to light up. Your body dashboard may light up with any of the following:

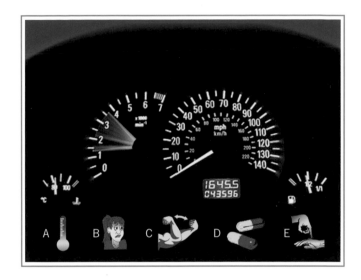

A: Temperature — You may feel more pain when it's cold out.

B: Stress chemicals — You may feel more pain when you are stressed or nervous.

C: Movement — Your movements may become sensitive – especially after surgery, injury or persistent pain.

D: Immunity — Your body may be more sensitive when you have the flu.

E: Pressure — You may be a lot more sensitive to pressure on your skin.

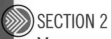

SECTION 2
Your nosy neighbors

When you develop pain in an area of your body and the nerves in the area "wake up," there are usually some interested neighbors.[5,6] Remember that your nervous system is connected, and it works like an alarm system. If the alarm in your house goes off, it probably wakes the neighbors right next to you. They are curious and concerned about you. If the alarm keeps going, some neighbors down the street may also wake up. Nerves work the same way. The areas in which you are experiencing pain have the alarm system going off all the time, and the tissues' neighbors have been awakened. It isn't uncommon to experience some sensitivity, such as aches and pains, or to sense a spreading pain.[19]

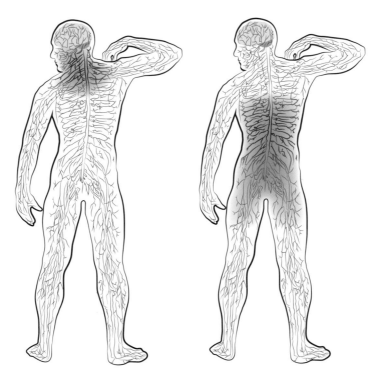

To add to this already irritable neighbor situation, the police are called to inspect the neighborhood. Your body contains various immune molecules traveling through your body to make sure you stay healthy. Think of immune molecules as little police officers checking out the neighborhood. With the alarms going off, the police officers are called to see if everything is OK. They will then go door-to-door, checking on all of the neighbors. This in itself will make the situation a little testier. With the police, or your immune molecules, checking in on the neighborhood, adjacent neighborhoods are also checked on, thus waking the other neighborhoods as well. This is all normal and expected. Agitated nerves may be felt as aches, but they may not indicate injury. It's important to note that previous crime areas in your body, such as old surgeries, scars and previously injured areas, will definitely be checked out by the police.

Remember there are nerve sensors that will sense the immune molecules. Old aches and pains may show up again, but it's due to sensitivity, not injury.

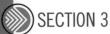

SECTION 3
Your body's Chief Executive Officer

All the areas in which you experience pain have extra-sensitive nerves. They need to send information somewhere, so something can be done. Nerves pass information on to the spinal cord, which in turn passes it on to the brain. This allows your brain to process the information and take action, such as stopping movement of a painful body part and going to see the doctor.[19]

When pain persists and there are many worries, the brain will analyze the incoming messages of danger very closely. A good way to think of this is when you press an X on your computer keyboard and four Xs show up on your screen instead. It's not the information you sent. Somehow, your computer overanalyzed your input on the computer keyboard, similar to placing a magnifying glass in the area.[7,20]

This response does not seem fair, but it's normal and essential to your survival. The already overactive nerve danger messages are amplified as it reaches the brain. The best description as to why this occurs would be to see your brain as the body's Chief Executive Officer (CEO).

Think of a large office building or organization.

At the top floor is the CEO running the organization. It's customary for each division of the company to provide the CEO with monthly reports.

Monthly reports, however, follow a line of command. The department manager

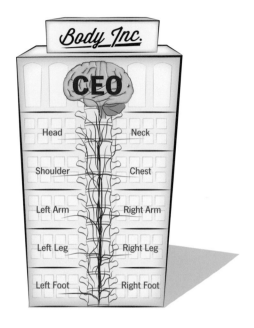

develops the report and then passes it on to the director who analyzes it and makes a few corrections if needed. Then he passes his version of the report on to the vice president. The vice president also checks the report, makes changes as needed and finally passes it on to the CEO.

What happens when there's a problem in a division? When a division of a company is under-performing, it's customary for a CEO to become worried.

The CEO now asks for weekly reports to find out what the issue is and to keep an eye on the department.

To ensure timely reports from the problem division, the CEO also informs the department manager to send the message straight to him/her, bypassing the director and vice president to speed up the communication process and allow for faster action.

Once enough information is gathered by the CEO, action is taken to correct the problem.

Nerves pass information on to the spinal cord, which in turn passes it on to the brain. This allows your brain to process the information and take action.

How does this pertain to your pain?

✓ Each of your body parts, such as your shoulders and hips, are divisions in the larger company called Body, Inc.

✓ Your body parts constantly send information to the brain to inform it of how they're doing.

✓ The information is sent to the brain, the CEO, via the nervous system and various checkpoints along the way, similar to how CEOs receive messages from managers, directors and vice presidents. En route, the message can become altered.

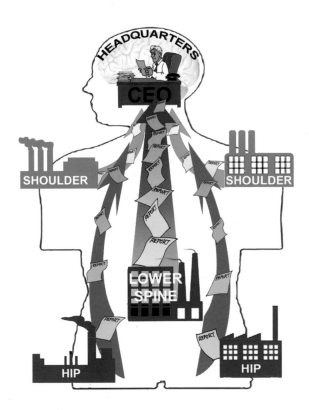

✓ If there's persistent pain in an area, the organizational process described previously is likely to occur.

As a result, more information will be sent to the brain.[21,22] When pain persists, extra-sensitive nerves cause increased messages to the spinal cord and ultimately to the brain to analyze. This is no fun, but again, a normal, protective process by your body to help you deal with the pain.

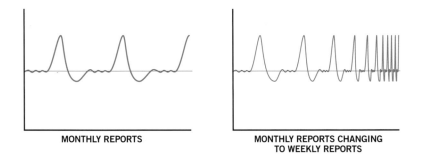

MONTHLY REPORTS   **MONTHLY REPORTS CHANGING TO WEEKLY REPORTS**

In the process, the messages to the brain will be less altered, and the brain will become more aware of the painful body part.

✓ A VERY IMPORTANT next step follows.

When the report finally arrives at the CEO's desk, it would make sense to carefully analyze all the data as if using a magnifying glass. This magnification has a protective job and is normal.

To add to the complexity, we need to remember that most CEOs are paranoid. Once the CEO is dealing with the troubled section, for example, the lower back, the CEO may start worrying about and snooping around in the other divisions, asking for more reports from them. Now the organization, which is you — Body, Inc. — becomes aware of all

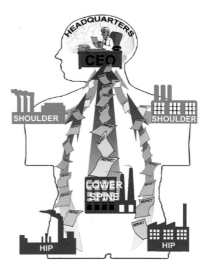

these areas. Compare this to the previous discussion of nosy neighbors and police officers knocking on doors.

Experiencing pain in other adjacent areas could be seen as normal and part of this survival process. It's not an indication of injury, but rather of sensitive nerves in the area and a CEO snooping around to make sure everything at Body, Inc. is OK.

CEO – Taking action

This all seems like gloom and doom, but there's some great news. If the CEO uncovers an issue, such as a nail in the foot, appropriate action is taken to resolve the issue, such as getting a tetanus shot, walking funny and putting on some shoes.

In many cases, however, the report reveals no real big issue – especially messages from tissues that have healed.

AS AN EXAMPLE, LET'S EXAMINE LOW BACK PAIN.
The back has been sore and painful for five years. Certainly there's been some injury, but tissues heal. The tissues are still sore, tired and sensitive. In this case, the lower-back division has been underperforming. The CEO, after analyzing the issue, realizes five people were gone this last month on leave and, in addition, five other people were on vacation, thus leaving the department a little short-handed. This is no big issue. They will all soon return and maybe undergo a quick human-resource policy change on the number of people per division that can leave at one time. In such a case, all is returned to normal with weekly reports changed back to monthly reports and all reports again sent to the CEO through the manager, director and vice president.

KNOWLEDGE CHANGED THE CEO'S RESPONSE.

Once pain patients become educated about the neuroscience of pain, they understand more about how danger messages are processed. Realizing that a lot of the pain they experience is due to extra-sensitive nerves, their nerve sensitivity is actually turned down.[8,9]

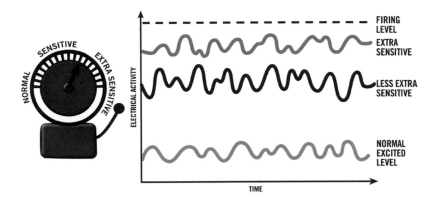

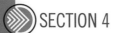
Your brain's board meetings and airline maps

The brain's processing of danger messages from the tissues is important in understanding your pain. For years, the belief was that there is a single pain area in the brain. When you stub your toe, the light bulb flashes on and there it is: pain. If pain

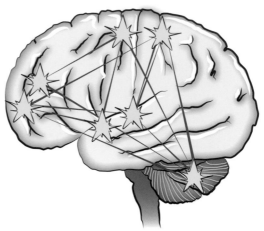

was so simple, it would be easy to remove this area, and all pain would be gone. When you have a pain experience, it is now well established by scientists that various areas of your brain are involved in processing this pain experience.[23,24] These areas then connect and form a pain map,[1,24,25] which covers all pain. Patients diagnosed with low-back pain, neck pain, fibromyalgia, chronic fatigue syndrome and more have very similar brain areas that are lit up. These areas were studied and documented as follows:

1. SENSATION AREA
Each body part, such as the back, neck, shoulder, hand or foot, is represented in body areas of the brain. These areas tell you where in your body you are experiencing sensations, including pain. Obviously, these areas are needed and, as a result, are active.

2. MOVEMENT AREA

The areas that plan, coordinate and execute your movements are also busy protecting you. Maybe some muscles needed to protect you stiffen up and do not allow you to bend as far forward.

3. FOCUS AND CONCENTRATION AREA

The areas dealing with focus and concentration are also busy dealing with your pain experience.

4. FEAR AREA

The emotional areas of the brain dealing with fear, such as fear of injury, re-injury or even fear of movement are called upon, especially when pain is poorly understood.

5. MEMORY AREA

The areas of the brain dealing with memory are busy. They remember previous similar experiences and call upon these strategies to help this time.

6. MOTIVATION AREA

The area dealing with motivation is now used to process pain, versus its job of motivating.

7. STRESS RESPONSE AREA

There are specialized areas in the brain dealing with stress. These centers control the release of various stress chemicals, such as adrenaline, into the body to help protect you. These centers also control sleep, body weight and body temperature.

Key issue

Various brain areas are involved in all pain experiences. These areas then communicate with each other to "discuss" the appropriate action. Think of this process as a board meeting.

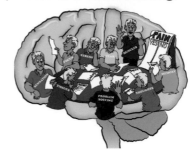

When danger messages are received from the tissue, the CEO calls for a board meeting to discuss the danger messages. If the board believes there is a threat and action is required, certain brain areas produce pain to protect you.

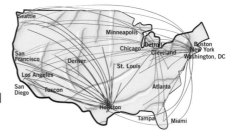

Another way to think of how the brain processes pain is an airline map. If you page through an airline magazine, you will notice the map showing where the airline flies.

With all the areas in your brain involved in a board meeting to process the danger messages, you have developed something similar to an airline map in the brain.

It's also important for you to know that, just as in real life, people fly different airlines. Each person who experiences pain uses the similar areas of the brain, but the pathways are different. Pain is individualized, which makes it so hard to treat.[2,26] You need treatment tailored to your pain.

A common, but unfortunate, saying is that pain is in your head. The saying implies that it's not real, but fabricated.[27] This is not true. However, pain is located in your head, within your brain. When you have pain, the brain is very active processing it. How your brain processes it determines the pain you experience. So, yes, your pain experience is in your head, but it's real. It can be measured, and it can be changed for the better.

Pain is individualized, which makes it so hard to treat.[2,26] You need treatment tailored to your pain.

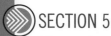 SECTION 5
Your body's injury —
ankle sprains and buses

To further explore how the brain processes danger, another common misbelief about pain signals from tissues needs to be dispelled. Many people are told or believe pain signals travel from an injured area and "tell" your brain there's pain. This is not true. All the tissues can "tell" the 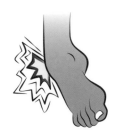 brain is that there is danger and something needs to be done.[2] For instance, examine an ankle sprain.

If you sprained your ankle right now, you would probably say that it hurts. Obviously.

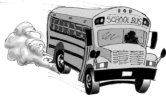 What happens if you sprain your ankle while you are crossing a busy road? As you roll your ankle, out of the corner of your eye you see a speeding school bus coming straight for you, and it's not stopping. Does the ankle still hurt? No, because you're too busy focusing on getting out of the way of the bus.

Ankles and all tissues in the body contain danger receptors, and all they do is alert the brain about dangers. If the ankle contained pain fibers, you would have experienced pain that may have caused you to fall down or move too slowly, thus threatening your life with the speeding bus coming toward you. Pain is a brain decision. In this case, it isn't logical for the brain to produce pain in the ankle. If you could listen in on the brain during such a decision-making situation, the brain would undoubtedly have to decide if a speeding bus is more dangerous than an ankle sprain. Can you think of times when you, or someone you know, had an injury, yet little or no pain?

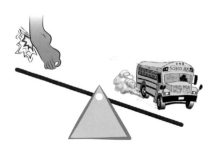

Pain is a decision by the brain, based on everything it knows about the threatening situation. In this case, the ankle sprain is not a threat and pain is not necessary to protect you until you successfully cross the road. Then an ankle sprain may be a big deal, causing the brain to produce pain.[1,2]

Many people with persistent pain have numerous concerns regarding their medical care, diagnosis and recovery. This leads to a big threat. Pain, called upon by the brain, is the logical defense.

BUT I'VE NEVER HAD AN INJURY; THE PAIN JUST STARTED!

Many people who read this and have persistent pain will say, "But I've never had an injury!"

- ✓ Tissue injury is not needed for pain.[2,28,29]
- ✓ Emotional stress can cause pain.[28,29]
- ✓ Many people suffering from pain had a time in their lives filled with many stressors, perhaps involving family, work or financial issues and even, unfortunately, abuse.[30]
- ✓ With all these stressors, the brain perceives threat and thus produces pain.

Your body under attack

Imagine yourself sitting at home watching TV, relaxing after a hard day of work. Your body systems are all in balance. Suddenly the door opens and a massive, roaring African lion enters the room.

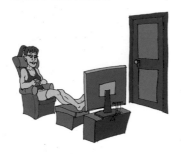

To deal with this immediate threat, your body systems will react to protect you, shifting the balance to prioritized tasks.[31] These systems include the following:

ADRENALINE[29]

Adrenaline is a stress chemical. It controls heart rate, breathing, blood flow, levels of alertness and more. In response to the threat of the lion, your heart rate increases rapidly to pump blood though

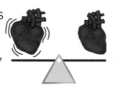
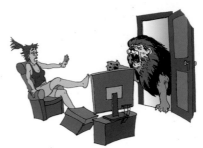
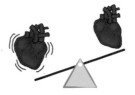
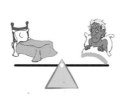
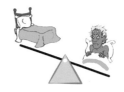

the body to areas needing blood and oxygen, such as your big muscles. Adrenaline causes you to be very alert. No time for a nap right now. Eyes wide open!

MUSCLES

In an immediate
threat response,
large muscles able to
help escape or fight
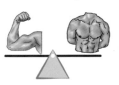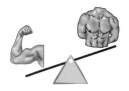
are needed, such as big, strong leg muscles for running away
and big arm muscles to punch the lion. Smaller postural or
abdominal muscles you have been working on in therapy
so diligently in the past are not needed right now. Shutting
down these muscles for the immediate threat seems like a
good strategy. They can be turned on when the threat has
been removed.[32]

STOMACH

Digestion of food
is slowed down or
even put on hold,
allowing for all
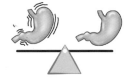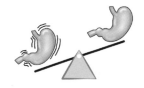
possible energy and blood flow to be directed to the immediate,
much-needed systems.[33]

LANGUAGE

When startled with a threat such as the lion, you might say a
few choice words, usually loudly and sharply.

BREATHING

With the threat, breathing becomes faster and shallower.

PAIN

Pain is a perception of threat. In this case, it would be a perception of greater 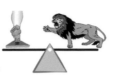 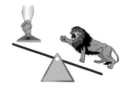 threat. If you stepped on a nail while running from the room, it would not be painful because the lion is a bigger threat.

HEALING

Your immune system helps you stay healthy and fight infections. This 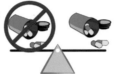 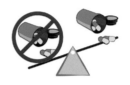 system is surely not immediately needed when a lion enters the room, so healing is slowed down. Your immune system can be resumed tomorrow if you are able to get away from the lion.[31,34]

INTIMACY

When a lion enters a room, sexual attraction and intimate thoughts are put on hold. 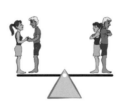 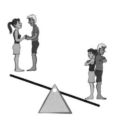 There is no time for intimacy; there are bigger issues.

OTHER

Other responses, such as lack of motivation and poor memory, also occur.

In the meantime, the local zookeeper shows up, captures the lion and removes the lion from the room. Your body systems, which have been all revved up, normalize and become balanced. They are ready to fight another day. Talk about feeling relieved and sinking into your seat! This process occurs daily as humans are faced with stressors. What a great system! This great system, however, is designed to elevate and calm – not run at high levels for prolonged periods.[31]

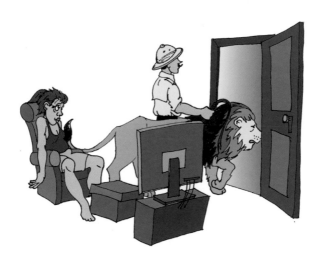

What does this have to do with me?

This is an interesting story, but how does it pertain to you and your pain? People who live in pain every day have a massive, roaring African lion following them around. The lion is a collection of the daily issues you face, 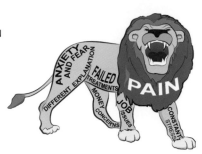 including pain, fear, anxiety, worries about work, money, failed treatments, different explanations for your pain and more. Clumped together, all these issues are a threat, similar to a close encounter with an African lion.

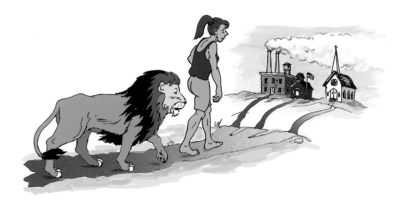

These systems, however, are designed to work for short periods to help you deal with a threat. People who have pain for long periods have this pain like a lion following them every day as they go to work, church, school and more.

This prolonged, protective response is very easily connected to many issues that pain patients deal with. The good news is that there is an explanation for this response, along with ways to cope, such as the following:

TENDER AREAS
With blood shifted away from areas, muscles and nerves become a lot more sensitive. They're not broken; they're just sensitive and sore.[35]

MOOD SWINGS
With increased stress, the body produces more stress chemicals, such as cortisol. It is now well known that if cortisol is altered long enough, mood swings occur.

APPETITE CHANGES
Cortisol changes appetite and food intake. Additionally, remember that many different areas of the brain are involved in processing pain. A key area, the hypothalamus, regulates hunger and affects food intake as well as changes in taste. It's also a key area to regulate body temperature.

FATIGUE
With stress and stress chemicals burning calories fast and furious, fatigue sets in.[34]

WEIGHT GAIN

Changes in cortisol are associated with increased weight gain. The hypothalamus that regulates appetite, hunger and a sense of being full is altered. Pain patients also move and exercise less. All of this can result in difficulty losing weight, which affects self-esteem.[36]

SLEEP DISTURBANCE

Stress chemicals make sleeping very hard – especially deep, restorative sleep. Processing pain also makes sleeping difficult. Body temperature is altered. The digestive system is altered. Sensitive tissues provide problematic positioning.[37]

POSTURE ISSUES

Strong, big muscles dominate. Smaller muscles dealing with posture have less blood supply and oxygen. The brain also questions the importance of posture in a survival situation.[38]

STOMACH SENSITIVITY

When under stress, blood is pulled away from the digestive system to protect big muscles. This makes the digestive system have to work double time, which makes it irritable.

LOW SEXUAL DRIVE

Reproduction is not needed when a lion enters the room. Over time, sexual drive and the hormones associated with reproduction, such as testosterone and estrogen, are altered. People in pain are less interested in such activities. Depression and self-awareness of the body and feeling less attractive also contribute to this issue.

PROBLEMS WITH FOCUS AND CONCENTRATION

Several studies have shown that cortisol alteration leads to problems with focus and concentration, especially for prolonged periods.

DEPRESSION

It is well established that altered cortisol, which is very prevalent in patients dealing with pain for prolonged periods, is a leading cause of depression.[14]

Given all the issues we have discussed, a bigger picture of your pain experience may start to look like this:

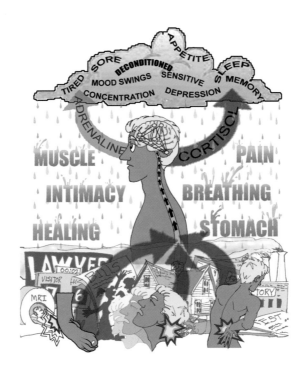

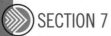

SECTION 7
Your treatment – taking back your life

Most likely, the main reason you are reading this book is to seek a way to eliminate your pain and get your life back. If you want to know how treatment can help, the preceding neuroscience information is important to understand. The focus will be on a few strategies that have shown to work really well with people struggling with persistent pain.

❶ KNOWLEDGE

Education is therapy. Gaining an understanding of the neuroscience of your pain will undoubtedly ease some fears, explain some unknowns and provide some hope. This alone will move you forward to recovery.[25,39] If you can start to understand that your pain is complex, how you think and process pain is vital to how much pain you experience, and that a big cause of your pain is heightened sensitivity, you are well on your way to recovery. In fact, studies have shown that your nerves will immediately start calming down when your awareness regarding the root of your pain increases. The drawings on the right, from brain-scan studies, show the difference before and after a 30-minute neuroscience education session, such as reading this book. The drawings from the scans show how the brain calms down.

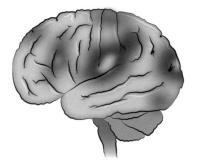
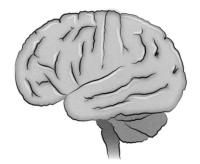

This newly gained knowledge of your pain, such as sensitive nerves and brain processing versus injured tissues, will have a calming effect on your extra-sensitive nerves. This is a sophisticated alarm system, and if you have been struggling for a prolonged period, it will only turn down a little bit at a time.[5,6]

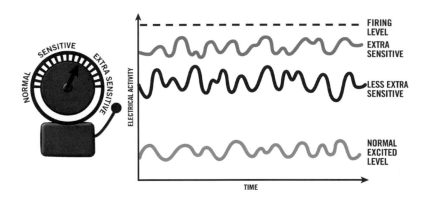

Another way to view how neuroscience education can help is to return to the African lion story.

We have already gone through the whole "what if a lion enters this room" scenario.

Now what would you do if, while watching TV after dinner and relaxing, a lion cub enters the room? Unless you have a major fear of lions, you'd be OK with it.
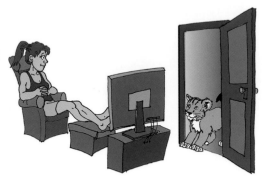
You may even go to the lion cub and pet it.

That's just it. If the threat can be made smaller, the body systems protecting it, such as adrenaline, cortisol or big muscles, are not needed. We believe being educated about your pain makes big lions smaller. You must develop a greater understanding of your pain. There is no need to make persistent pain this unknown, big, threatening African lion in your life.

Many people with persistent pain…

✓ Climb mountains
✓ Run marathons
✓ Work as CEOs
✓ Go back to school to complete a degree
✓ Start a business
✓ Volunteer their services to the community

❷ AEROBIC EXERCISE

Research has shown that aerobic exercise, which gets your heart pumping a little faster and pumps blood and oxygen through your body, helps calm nerves down.[40,41]

Don't worry; no need to run marathons or climb mountains.

Studies have shown that brisk walking – between 10-20 minutes – is all that is needed to have a calming effect on nerves. In fact, most people can easily get there just by raising their heart rate 20 beats a minute.[42] Also remember that if you pump blood and oxygen through your body regularly, you will achieve the following benefits:

✓ Less muscle soreness and fatigue
✓ Better sleep
✓ More enjoyment of the taste of food
✓ Weight loss
✓ Decreased stress levels
✓ Fewer mood swings
✓ Decreased or no depression

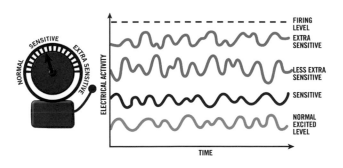

Helpful exercise strategies

There are many strategies you can try to help you exercise and calm down. In fact, books have been written just about that. Here are some helpful strategies people have used over the years.

> **Start small:** Start with three to four minutes of exercise. Every two days, add a minute until you reach 15-20 minutes of regular exercise. Walking is an easy option. You can substitute walking with biking or swimming. Remember: increasing your heart rate is the main goal.

> **Make a plan:** On paper, write down a plan that includes where you will be exercising, at what time and for how long.

> **Rest:** Don't exercise every day. Schedule days off. We suggest working out five days a week.

> **Get a partner:** Exercise with a friend, neighbor or family member. Explain your plan so they can help.

> **Back off:** Many people in pain are doing too much exercise. Pace yourself.

> **Ready the words:** If you experience some aches and pains while exercising, remind yourself that you are sensitive and all is well. Your tissues are tired, sensitive and sore; you are working on making them healthier.

> **Get away:** Avoid working out at home. Get outside in the fresh air. If it's cold, go walk in the mall. Home is usually filled with stressful issues, such as housework and family needs.

> **Log your progress:** Start a log book or journal. After each workout, write what you did. Record some positive thoughts about your workout, your day and your progress.

> **Set a goal:** Be specific. It may be to complete a loop around the park or charity walk by a certain date. Plan and prepare.

> **Breathe:** When you exercise, remember to breathe. It's amazing to see how many people don't. Take nice big breaths. The mixture of blood and oxygen flushing through your body will help calm the nerves and excite the brain.

❸ MEDICINE

First, all questions about your medication should be directed to your doctor. With all your medical experiences, you are probably aware that pharmaceutical companies have developed a series of drugs to calm nerves down. Skillful delivery of medication may be helpful for some patients – especially those more affected on the severe scale.

Did you know the brain produces the most potent pain medicine on the planet, helping people survive severe injuries while experiencing little or no pain?[20] The brain produces these "happy chemicals" that then have a calming effect and change the danger messages. This scenario is described as a "wet brain." It's juicy and full of good, healthy medicine, which is able to be released to help you when you're in pain, like stubbing a toe. People with persistent pain have "dry brains," where the medicine is dried up to make you more sensitive to protect yourself.[5,6]

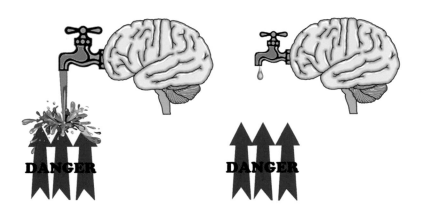

Unfortunately, people who have struggled with pain for a long time have this drug cabinet affected in a negative way. As the brain becomes more worried and interested in what's going on in the low back, it – in essence – takes the numbing medicine out of the body, making you more sensitive to protect yourself. This is one reason why you have developed some increased sensitivity for tasks that were not painful in the past.

When experiencing persistent pain, your brain produces less of the medicine helping you on a daily basis to deal with pain. Is this permanent? Can it be changed? The answer is yes. It can be changed as follows:

KNOWLEDGE
Increased knowledge of your pain experience allows for greater understanding and less fear. With less fear and a greater realistic understanding of a pain experience, the brain will once again produce increased numbing medicine to help.

AEROBIC EXERCISE
After approximately 10 minutes of moderate aerobic exercise, the brain produces more of a calming effect on nerves. Pumping blood and oxygen around nerves also calms them down.

MEDICINE
Low-dose anti-depressants are able to gently open this medicine cabinet in the brain.

FOODS
Foods high in carbohydrates, such as bread and pasta, help produce a calming effect. Carbohydrates contain tryptophan, which is turned into calming medicine in the brain.[43]

❹ SLEEP HYGIENE

Few things have as huge an effect on our health as sleep. At least eight hours of sleep is needed for most people. Americans average six hours a night and people in pain average less. Even if you sleep a lot, you never feel refreshed when you wake.

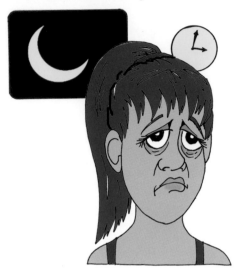

Sleep deprivation has been linked to increased rates of pain, obesity, depression and other health-related disorders. Changing sleep habits is hard, but important for your recovery.

There are many sleep strategies, including the following:

SHUT OFF

Shut the lights, television and computer off because they stimulate your nervous system and brain.

SET TIME

Have a set time to go to bed. It has been shown that the more time you sleep before midnight, the more refreshed you are in the morning.

NAPS

If you sleep in the day for more than a 20-minute nap, it will have a negative effect on your much-needed night's sleep. If you need a nap or two, make them power naps of 20 minutes or fewer.

CAFFEINE
Don't consume caffeine late in the afternoon or evening.

NOTES
Park your ideas. When you have a lot of things on your mind, write them down so your brain can go to sleep.

DARK AND COOL
Darken and cool your bedroom.

BED BUDDIES
No kids or animals in your bed.

ALCOHOL
Limit alcohol in the evening to avoid bathroom breaks in the middle of the night when you need the deep, resting phases of sleep.

WATER
Limit water intake in the evening to avoid bathroom breaks.

CLOSE YOUR EYES
Force yourself to sleep and not wake in the morning. After doing this for a few days, these closed-eye sessions will transfer into sleep.

EXERCISE
You sleep better when you exercise regularly.

❺ GOALS AND PACING

Many people in pain have no goals. They may be thinking, "How can I set goals if I can barely get up in the morning and get through the day?" Many other people in pain have goals, but they are so big, they seem out of reach and not even worth a try. For example, a goal may be to clean the house, but given all the tasks, such as washing, dusting and vacuuming, the task is daunting and will no doubt cause pain.

Any task can be broken down into smaller parts. The following is an example:

> Think about cleaning the house. In itself, the task is huge. Make a list of tasks associated with cleaning the house. For example, vacuum, dust, mop, etc. Once you have the list, choose the one you would really like to do. If your goal is to vacuum, for example, count the rooms needing vacuuming. Once you have the number, make a priority list. If you could only vacuum one room, which one would it be? That room is A, the next B and then C, D and E. Now, based on your pain and your newfound knowledge, determine how much of a room you would be able to vacuum before putting the vacuum away, with enough energy remaining to get through your day.

For example, you may think half of a room is your limit. Now we divide the rooms into A1, A2, B1, B2, etc. Before your eyes, you have an attainable goal of vacuuming your house. Sure, it may take 10 days, but it may be the first time in months or years you've vacuumed. As you get healthier, A1 and A2 are combined, and now you vacuum the house in five days. All tasks can be broken down. Similarly, meals don't have to be cooked in one session. They can steadily be prepared throughout one or more days. Not all vegetables need to be cut up at once. Not all laundry has to be done in one session. Not all e-mails have to be answered in one session and so forth.

WHEN MAKING A GOAL LIST, CONSIDER THE FOLLOWING:

✓ **The things you need to do,** such as cooking and cleaning. Find ways to break these chores down into manageable pieces.

✓ **The things you would love to do.** Most people are shocked when told that there is probably no reason you cannot get back to _____ (fill in your dream). This includes dancing, running a marathon, hosting Thanksgiving, etc. Sure, it will take time, but walking a half mile quickly translates to a mile, followed by run/walking a mile and a half and then completing a 5K race and so on. Remember: goal setting is one part. As you gain knowledge of your pain, empower yourself, get healthier and sleep better, these tasks get easier. Dream big, take your time and keep moving forward – even if it's small steps.

CONCLUSION

The choice is yours. The information presented here is based on thousands of research studies and personal stories. Regardless of the best medicine, education session or personal coaching, the decision is ultimately yours. It's easy to read a little book on pain, but now you have a goal. There's no time like the present to apply what you've learned to treat your pain, so you can begin to move on with your life. Remember that pain is normal. Living in pain is not.

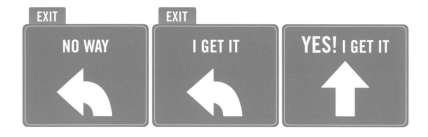

Scientific support for your recovery

1. Moseley GL. A pain neuromatrix approach to patients with chronic pain. *Man Ther.* Aug 2003;8(3):130-140.
2. Moseley GL. Reconceptualising pain according to modern pain sciences. *Physical Therapy Reviews.* 2007;12:169-178.
3. Haldeman S. Presidential address, North American Spine Society: Failure of the pathology model to predict back pain. *Spine.* 1990;15(7):718-724.
4. Louw A, Butler DS. Chronic Pain. In: S.B. B, Manske R, eds. *Clinical Orthopaedic Rehabilitation.* 3rd Edition ed. Philadelphia, PA: Elsevier; 2011.
5. Louw A. *Your Nerves Are Having Back Surgery.* Minneapolis: OPTP; 2012.
6. Louw A. *Whiplash: An Alarming Message from your Nerves.* Minneapolis: OPTP; 2012.
7. Butler DS. *The Sensitive Nervous System.* Adelaide: Noigroup; 2000.
8. Louw A, Diener I, Butler DS, Puentedura EJ. The effect of neuroscience education on pain, disability, anxiety, and stress in chronic musculoskeletal pain. *Archives of physical medicine and rehabilitation.* Dec 2011;92(12):2041-2056.
9. Louw A, Puentedura EL, Mintken P. Use of an abbreviated neuroscience education approach in the treatment of chronic low back pain: A case report. *Physiotherapy theory and practice.* Jul 3 2011.
10. Moseley GL, Hodges PW, Nicholas MK. A randomized controlled trial of intensive neurophysiology education in chronic low back pain. *Clinical Journal of Pain.* 2004;20:324-330.
11. Moseley GL. Unravelling the barriers to reconceptualisation of the problem in chronic pain: the actual and perceived ability of patients and health professionals to understand the neurophysiology. *J Pain.* 2003;4(4):184-189.
12. Barker RA, Barasi S. *Neuroscience at a Glance.* Oxford: Blackwell; 1999.
13. Lundy-Ekman L. Neuroscience. *Fundamentals for Rehabilitation.* Philadelphia: WB Saunders; 1998.
14. Smart KM, Blake C, Staines A, Doody C. Self-reported pain severity, quality of life, disability, anxiety and depression in patients classified with 'nociceptive,' 'peripheral neuropathic' and 'central sensitisation' pain. The discriminant validity of mechanisms-based classifications of low back (+/-leg) pain. *Manual therapy.* Apr 2012;17(2):119-125.
15. Kendall NAS, Linton SJ, Main CJ. *Guide to assessing psychosocial yellow flags in acute low back pain: risk factors for long term disability and work loss.* Wellington: Accident Rehabilitation & Compensation Insurance Corporation of New Zealand and the National Health Committee; 1997.
16. Waddell G, Newton M, Henderson I, al. e. A fear-avoidance beliefs questionnaire (FABQ) and the role of fear avoidance beliefs in chronic low back pain and disability pain. 1993;52:157-168.
17. Devor M. Sodium channels and mechanisms of neuropathic pain. *J Pain.* Jan 2006;7(1 Suppl 1):S3-S12.
18. Devor M. The pathophysiology of damaged peripheral nerves. In: Wall PD, Melzack R, eds. *Textbook of Pain.* 3rd ed. Edinburgh: Churchill Livingstone; 1994.
19. Gifford LS. Pain, the tissues and the nervous system. *Physiotherapy.* 1998;84:27-33.
20. Butler D, Moseley G. *Explain Pain.* Adelaide: Noigroup; 2003.
21. Woolf CJ, Salter MW. Neuronal plasticity: increasing the gain in pain. *Science.* Jun 9 2000;288(5472):1765-1769.
22. Woolf CJ. Central sensitization: uncovering the relation between pain and plasticity. *Anesthesiology.* Apr 2007;106(4):864-867.

23. Doidge N. *The Brain That Changes Itself.* New York: Penguin Books; 2007.
24. Puentedura EJ, Louw A. A neuroscience approach to managing athletes with low back pain. *Phys Ther Sport.* Aug 2012;13(3):123-133.
25. Moseley GL. Widespread brain activity during an abdominal task markedly reduced after pain physiology education: fMRI evaluation of a single patient with chronic low back pain. *Aust J Physiother.* 2005;51(1):49-52.
26. Moseley GL. Joining forces – combining cognition-targeted motor control training with group or individual pain physiology education: a successful treatment for chronic low back pain. *J Man Manip Therap.* 2003;11(2):88-94.
27. Melzack R. Pain and the neuromatrix in the brain. *J Dent Educ.* 2001;65: 1378-1382.
28. Merskey H, Bogduk N. *Classification of Chronic Pain.* 2nd ed. Seattle: IASP Press; 1994.
29. Riva R, Mork PJ, Westgaard RH, Okkenhaug Johansen T, Lundberg U. Catecholamines and heart rate in female fibromyalgia patients. *Journal of Psychosomatic Research.* Jan 2012;72(1):51-57.
30. Hauser W, Kosseva M, Uceyler N, Klose P, Sommer C. Emotional, physical, and sexual abuse in fibromyalgia syndrome: a systematic review with meta-analysis. *Arthritis Care Res (Hoboken).* Jun 2011;63(6):808-820.
31. Sapolsky RM. *Why zebras don't get ulcers: an updated guide to stress, stress-related diseases, and coping.* New York: W.H. Freeman and Co; 1998.
32. Hodges PW, Moseley GL. Pain and motor control of the lumbopelvic region: effect and possible mechanisms. *J Electromyogr Kinesiol.* Aug 2003;13(4): 361-370.
33. Goldenberg DL. Diagnosis and differential diagnosis of fibromyalgia. *The American Journal of Medicine.* Dec 2009;122(12 Suppl):S14-21.
34. Nijs J, Meeus M, Van Oosterwijck J, et al. In the mind or in the brain? Scientific evidence for central sensitisation in chronic fatigue syndrome. *Eur J Clin Invest.* Feb 2012;42(2):203-212.
35. Fernandez-Carnero J, Fernandez-de-las-Penas C, de la Llave-Rincon AI, Ge HY, Arendt-Nielsen L. Bilateral myofascial trigger points in the forearm muscles in patients with chronic unilateral lateral epicondylalgia: a blinded, controlled study. *Clin J Pain.* Nov-Dec 2008;24(9):802-807.
36. Riva R, Mork PJ, Westgaard RH, Lundberg U. Comparison of the cortisol awakening response in women with shoulder and neck pain and women with fibromyalgia. *Psychoneuroendocrinology.* Feb 2012;37(2):299-306.
37. Mork PJ, Nilsen TI. Sleep problems and risk of fibromyalgia: longitudinal data on an adult female population in Norway. *Arthritis Rheum.* Jan 2012;64(1):281-284.
38. Edmondston S, Bjornsdottir G, Palsson T, Solgard H, Ussing K, Allison G. Endurance and fatigue characteristics of the neck flexor and extensor muscles during isometric tests in patients with postural neck pain. *Manual therapy.* Aug 2011;16(4):332-338.
39. Moseley L. Combined physiotherapy and education is efficacious for chronic low back pain. *Aust J Physiother.* 2002;48(4):297-302.
40. Busch AJ, Barber KA, Overend TJ, Peloso PM, Schachter CL. Exercise for treating fibromyalgia syndrome. *Cochrane Database Syst Rev.* 2007(4):CD003786.
41. Kuphal KE, Fibuch EE, Taylor BK. Extended swimming exercise reduces inflammatory and peripheral neuropathic pain in rodents. *J Pain.* Dec 2007;8(12):989-997.
42. Hoffman MD, Shepanski MA, Mackenzie SP, Clifford PS. Experimentally induced pain perception is acutely reduced by aerobic exercise in people with chronic low back pain. *J Rehabil Res Dev.* Mar-Apr 2005;42(2):183-190.
43. Barnard N. *Foods That Fight Pain.* New York: Three Rivers Press; 1998.

More patient books by Adriaan Louw

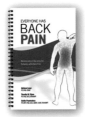

Everyone Has Back Pain
Understand how pain truly works in the body and discover simple, easy-to-apply strategies to calm your nerves and lessen your back pain.

ITEM #8754

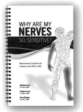

Why Are My Nerves So Sensitive?
Treat CRPS (or RSD) by first addressing the brain — the source of all pain. Only then will you find success treating the tissues.

ITEM #8752

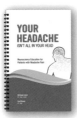

Your Headache Isn't All In Your Head
Uncover what's causing your persistent headaches, understand how pain really works and learn how you can alleviate or prevent your headache pain.

ITEM #8749

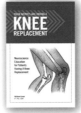

Your Nerves Are Having a Knee Replacement
Learn how the body and its nervous system react to a knee replacement in order to effectively calm your nerves and reduce knee pain.

ITEM #8753

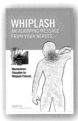

Whiplash: An Alarming Message from Your Nerves
Learn how your nerves become sensitive after a whiplash injury, how to ease the pain and why early, gentle movement is important for recovery.

ITEM #8744

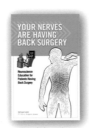

Your Nerves Are Having Back Surgery
Discover what your nervous system experiences when you undergo back surgery — why nerve sensitization occurs and how you can calm it down.

ITEM #8745

Available at OPTP.com

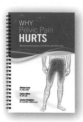

Why Pelvic Pain Hurts
Weave through the stigma and complexities of chronic pelvic pain to discover what's causing your pain and start your journey to recovery.

ITEM #8742

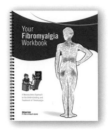

Your Fibromyalgia Workbook
Turn down your extra-sensitive nervous system. Understanding your pain lets you hurt less, do more and recover from fibromyalgia symptoms.

ITEM #8747

Clinical Resources by Adriaan Louw

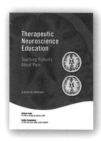

Therapeutic Neuroscience Education: Teaching Patients About Pain; A Guide for Clinicians
Master neuroscience education with this classic text. Adriaan Louw teams up with Emilio Puentedura to deliver an evidence-based perspective on how the body and brain collaborate to create pain, how to convey this view to patients and how to integrate therapeutic neuroscience education into a practice.

ITEM #8748

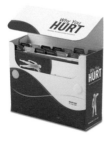

Why You Hurt: Therapeutic Neuroscience Education System
Discover the ultimate neuroscience teaching tool. This comprehensive system includes 120+ full-color, two-sided education cards with teaching cues and scientific support, 50 reproducible and downloadable homework cards, 12 pain questionnaire cards, detailed instructions, discussion of TNE and a teaching index.

ITEM #8751

Available at OPTP.com